Stay Thin For]

by Rachel Henderson

Contents

Contents 2

Introduction...3

Why Diets Do Not Work 4

How All Diets are Alike 6

Making Changes 7

A Healthy Balanced Diet 8

How Often To Eat...14

What To Eat 16

What to Drink 18

Listening to Your Body 20

How To Move Forward 23

Exercising 25

Eating 27

Action Plan..29

Eating and Stress...33

Weight and sleep...34

Weight and the Weather..36

Getting Support...37

Your Family 38

Temptation 39

Positive Thinking 40

Conclusion 42

Introduction

There are masses of diet books on the market. They are also all sorts of diets that people can try. They tend to change with different trends. Perhaps a celebrity does one and that becomes popular or there is a best selling book with the diet in.

The diets and books all have one thing in common. There is a person, who has lost lots of weight using the technique who comes up with a fantastic story about how they had tried many diets and none had worked before and this one did. It always makes everyone who has had the same experience feel that this one will work for them.

The problem is that we never know how long it works for. Most diets work well to start with, some people even reach their target weight. But what happens a few years down the line, do they keep the weight off. A few people will, but statistically, most people do not. Most people slip back in to bad habits and put weight back on, often more than they lost.

This book is not about faddy diets and losing weight in the short term. It is about changing your lifestyle so that you do not ever get overweight again. You will need to change your eating habits, the way you exercise and your attitude towards food and yourself. It will not be easy, but it will give rewards that will last a lifetime, rather than a short time.

Why Diets Do Not Work

There are all sorts of diets, but none of them work. They are all based around restricting you to certain foods, low calories or things like this. These are not sustainable over the long term.

Having a low amount of calories can make you crave foods. It can also make you feel deprived and you may decide that you deserve those unhealthy foods that taste so good and it could be a turn around which sets you back to putting on weight again. You may be on a diet that restricts the types of food you can eat, so you can only eat apples, for example. This can only be done for the short term before your body demands different types of food.

If we restrict what we are eating, then our body thinks that we are starving ourselves. It will hold on to every bit of fat that it can, because naturally it needs to keep it just in case there is a time of famine. Before we had such convenient lifestyles, food was not always readily available. It was natural for the body to make us crave high energy and high fat foods to give us a quick energy burst and also to store up fat reserves. Our body also needs certain nutrients and if we are not getting those, because of a restricted diet we will find we crave foods or get unwell.

We need to understand that our bodies have particular nutritional needs. The government provide us with guidelines on these and we can also get the information from the doctor. The food pyramid is often used as a way of illustrating what should be eating and in what quantities.

Fruit and vegetables should be eaten in large quantities, followed by carbohydrates such as bread, pasta, rice, cereals and potatoes, then proteins such as fish, meat and beans. A small amount of fats and oils are required and water is required in large quantities.

Stay Thin For Life by Rachel Henderson

This is all very well, but our foods are often sold in packages combining different nutrients and so it can be difficult to know whether you are getting enough. Also many foods that we can buy are too full of fat, sugar and salt which cause us to gain weight easily. Even many diet foods are packed full of unhealthy ingredients and the wording on packaging is often misleading.

Therefore it is important to learn a lot more about foods for ourselves. Understand what is healthy and what is not and do not take anyone else's word for it.

How All Diets are Alike

Although diets do differ a lot in the advice you are given in what to eat, there are some similarities between them. The main one is that they all restrict your calorie intake.

You may not agree, but in the end they do all end up in people eating less calories. This is obviously with any calorie controlled diet as the whole point is to count calories and therefore reduce them. However, even diets where you can eat all you want, end up in people eating less calories. This is an unconscious thing and there are a number of reasons. In a low fat diet, you are eliminating a high calorie food group and so are likely to eat less calories. In a low carbohydrate diet, you are again eliminate a high calorie food group. You are also restricted in the types of food that you can eat. Therefore with less choice, you will eat less. This is because naturally we like choice. It is good for us to have a variety to our diet and that is why we don't want to eat the same thing all of the time. This has been shown in the way that people tend to eat more when there are lots of different things to eat, such as at a buffet. In restricting the amount of foods that we have to choose from, it means that we will eat less and therefore lose weight.

Most diets also recommend increasing exercise. This burns off calories and help with burning fat as well and therefore is something which should help everyone to lose weight.

Therefore, it probably doesn't matter which one you choose, you will be likely to lose some weight, as long as you stick to it. But will you be able to stick to it and if so, how long for?

Making Changes

If you want to lose weight and then keep it off, you will need to make changes to your life, changes which you will have to commit to doing for your whole life.

This means that you do not decide to cut out chocolate for a week or a month, but you decide to make a change for your whole life. This means that you need to make changes that are sustainable.

You want to be able to know, in your head that you are being honest with yourself. Do not decide that you will give up chocolate for life, when you know that at certain times of the month you crave it and cannot stop yourself eating it. Think of things that will be more manageable.

A good place to start is to keep a food diary for a few weeks. Write down everything that you eat and any exercise that you do. Be completely honest because it will only be you looking at it. You can then start to look at things that you can change in your diet and where you might need to increase your exercise. You will need to know about healthy eating and exercise though, or else you will not know what you are doing right and what you are doing wrong.

A Healthy Balanced Diet

The government recommend that we all eat a healthy balanced diet. If we do so, then we should get all the nutrients we need to keep our body in top condition and we should be an ideal weight. However, there are many people that do not know what is meant by a healthy diet or others that think they know, but actually do not. It is well worth checking to make sure that you fully understand what a healthy diet is.

Fruit and Vegetables

We often hear about having '5-a-day'. This is the optimum amount of fruit and vegetables to have, but it is important to know exactly what this refers to. Firstly, you need to know that this is a minimum amount. The actual recommendation is 2-3 fruit and 3-5 vegetables a day. This is not just 5 different items, but also the correct amount of each item. A portion of fruit and vegetables, generally refers to an amount the size of your fist. The exception is dried fruit where the fact that they are dehydrated means they are smaller. Therefore three dried apricots would be a portion of fruit or a tablespoon of sultanas or raisins.

It is important to have a good variety of fruit and vegetables because they are nutrient rich, but do not all contain the same nutrients. They all contain vitamin C which can be leached out during the cooking process, however, cabbage and onions are easier to digest when they are cooked and cooking carrots and tomatoes actually helps release some of the nutrients they contain. It is therefore worth having a mixture of cooked and uncooked vegetables.

Fruit and vegetables are seen as a great food if you are trying to lose weight because they are low in calories. This is true of vegetables, but some fruits can be high in calories because they are high in sugar. Although they contain no fat, the fruit sugar can easily be turned in to fat by the body and so it is important to not only make sure that you do not overeat when it comes to fruit, but also eat less of the highly sugary types such as grapes, melon and dried fruits.

Some people find it difficult to get enough portions of fruit and vegetables. However, if you spread them through the day, it can really help. A drink of fruit juice can be a good start, adding a sprinkle of sultanas or other dried fruit on to cereal or having an apple, pear or banana as a between meal snack or instead of a pudding. You can have some tomatoes with your lunch or in your sandwich. Vegetables are often more difficult for people. Some people think they do not like vegetables and find it hard to include enough with their meals.

Make sure that you do not only have vegetables with your main cooked meal but also with your other one. You could have vegetable soup or salad with a sandwich. You could put some salad in with your sandwich filling or have some carrot sticks, cucumber slices or celery with it. You could even have a small salad or some crudities as a between meal snack.

With your main meal, you can blend vegetables to make a sauce, add extra vegetables in to pasta dishes, as toppings on pizza or in with meat dishes. You do not have to have them plain, but have sauces on them to make them more exciting. Experiment with different way of cooking them. Roasted vegetables can be very tasty, as can stir fry. Some are delicious steamed. It all depends on the specific vegetable and how much you like the taste. It is worth trying different types, maybe things that you thought you do not like. Cook them in different ways, find some new recipes which incorporate them.

Many recipes and dishes do not have enough vegetables in them. This can be true you buy a ready meal and when you follow a recipe. However, it is easy to add your own, by perhaps having a salad with the meal or putting some peas and beans in with a curry for example. Eating out can be more difficult and you may need to ask for a side salad or bowl of vegetables with your meal when you order. You can get really inventive, when you start thinking about it and you can soon easily incorporate enough fruit and vegetables in to your daily meals.

Carbohydrates

All countries tend to have a staple carbohydrate which forms part of many meals. In India that is rice, in Ireland it is potatoes, in England it is bread and in China it is rice. Carbohydrates give us energy and they are foods which either contain sugar or complex sugars which the body breaks down to its simplest state in order to use for fuel. Fruits and vegetables contain sugars too and are a source of carbohydrate.

Carbohydrates such as white rice, white flour, white pastry, potatoes and white pasta are other processed cereals very easy for the body to break down. This is not good for a number of reasons. Firstly the energy is released quickly and we can tend to want other food soon after eating it because we need more energy. It also does not fill us up that much and so we are soon hungry again.

Having carbohydrates which are not so processed, such as oats, wholemeal pasta and bread and brown rice feel more bulky in the stomach and stop you feeling hungry so soon. They are also harder to break down, which means that the sugars are released more slowly, so the energy is released at a gentler rate and lasts for longer. It is therefore good to try to replace these white foods with wholegrain ones. It should stop us eating as much and help to keep the weight down. The white and sugary carbohydrates also seem to make you want more and more of them. It is not know why, but it is a good reason not to eat them. There is a recommendation that we have two portions of wholegrain a day. This is because it has a good fibre content. The fibre is good for cleansing the body and it also fills us up.

Protein

Protein does many good things in the body including helping to build muscle and form cells. There are a selection of different types of protein and we need all of them. All forms can be found in meat and fish, eggs and dairy. Vegetarian sources such as beans, lentils, nuts, seeds, grains and soya products will provide all the necessary proteins as long as they are eaten in combination with each other.

Many sources of protein are high in fat, such as eggs and meat. Therefore it is important to try to limit how much you eat. In the UK most people get more than enough protein in their diet and so it should not be a problem.

Many people think that protein is useful in building muscle and take protein shakes when they are working out. Although they are good when you want to bulk up, once you have completed that part of your exercise, you will find that protein is not necessary. Your body can only use so much in a day and it will not use the rest, so you could be wasting your time and money.

Fats and Oils

Fats and Oils include any sort of cooking oil as well as hard fats like butter, lard and margarine. We do need a certain amount of fat in the body, it helps protect the organs and keeps us warm. However, too much fat can be harmful and many of us do tend to have too much.

There are many hidden fats in foods, which perhaps mean that we are eating more than we realise. There is fat in meat, fish and dairy products. There is fat in pastries, cakes and biscuits. There are also fats in take aways and ready meals. We tend to get enough fat in our diet without adding extra when we are cooking or spreading it on our bread. It is important to therefore make sure that you understand how much fat is in foods and note how much you are having.

Low fat foods can be not as good as they seem. If a food just has less fat in than other equivalents, then this is great. However, if it has the fat replaced with sugars and additives, then this may not be so good. It could be better to just eat less of the food, rather than replace it with something which has all sorts of chemicals in.

It is also worth being very wary about things that say they have low fat. They could be products that are naturally low in fat anyway or they may only have a small percentage less fat and this may not be much different to the full fat equivalent. Check the calories of the food and compare it to equivalent higher fat products and see what calorie saving you actually make.

Balancing it All

The government recommendation is that people have half a plate of vegetables per meal, a quarter of a plate of protein and a quarter of a plate of carbohydrates. This is quite a rough guide but it can be a lot easier than weighing foods and calculating the exact amount of nutrients in it. There could be computer programs or websites that will do this for you, but it is not really necessary.

The point of having a varied diet is that you have a good range of different things to eat and so you should get all the nutrients that you need. This actually can be very easy to do, but it can be making sure the quantities are right or that you do not have too many unhealthy things between meals that is important. It is also important to do regular exercise as well.

It is worth bearing in mind, that it is possible to get all the necessary nutrients but still be unhealthy because you are eating all sorts of unhealthy foods as well or eating too much. Therefore quantity is important and make sure you do not use too big a plate or pile it too high.

How Often To Eat

An old fashioned approach to eating is to have just three meals a day. Have breakfast, something at lunchtime and then an evening meal. However, research has shown that this may not be such a good approach for all people.

These days many people skip breakfast, thinking that it will help them to be healthier. The problem is that if you are really hungry when it comes to mealtime, then you have a tendency to eat more. So when it comes to lunch time, you will eat an enormous meal or you will have unhealthy snacks beforehand. This means that it is far better to eat little and often, as long as you are eating healthy things.

It is much more natural for mammals to graze at their food. We are often told that this is not the way to be. If we graze all day and have big meals, then this will put on weight. But if we do not have meals and just graze, then it could be healthier for us. However, in reality this is not a practical thing to do.

It can be much better to have three main meals, which are not that big and then small snacks in between. This could mean something like a small bowl of cereal for breakfast, some fruit mid morning, a small salad and sandwich for lunch, a few nuts in the afternoon, a cooked meal and then a slice of toast in the evening. This should keep hunger at bay, but not mean that we have so much to eat that we put on weight.

This may seem like a lot of food, but as long as you keep your meals small, then you can eat this much and still maintain a healthy weight, especially if you make sure that you exercise as well.

Problems come when you snack between meals on crisps and

chocolate, have take aways and eat out for your main meals or have huge portions. It can also be a problem if you eat foods high in fat and sugar so go easy on those as well.

What To Eat

With the information about nutrition, you should be able to start to get an idea of what sorts of things you should be eating.

For breakfast it is a good idea to have a wholegrain cereal, poached egg on wholegrain toast or fruit and yoghurt. Porridge is great, as is any cereal with very little sugar added. You may find that you will have to make your own muesli or granola to keep it healthy enough, but there are some cereals that do have a low sugar content. Fruit juice can be a good addition as well. However, if you often get hungry when you reduce your portion sizes, then have fruit instead of juice because it will you up more than just having a liquid.

Mid morning it can be a good idea to have a piece of fruit.

For lunch have wholegrain bread with a low fat protein such as grilled chicken or ham and some salad, whether in the sandwich or on the side. Either that or have some vegetable soup, it is a good way to get a portion of vegetables. You could also have beans of toast or a roasted vegetable and ham toastie. If you had egg on toast for breakfast and do not feel like bread again, you could even have have cereal.

In the afternoon we can often get a bit of a slump. It is a good idea to have some nuts or seeds. Choose the unsalted variety and do not have too many, half a handful should be plenty. You can have sultanas or dried apricots with them if you wish, but again not too many, just 3 dried apricots or a tablespoon of sultanas.

The evening meal should be carefully balanced, with half a plate of vegetables, a variety each day, a quarter of a plate of low fat protein such as fish, meat, beans or lentils and a quarter of a plate of carbohydrate such as rice, pasta or potatoes. You can have

16

gravy or sauce on the meal, but try to avoid having cheese or white sauce, which tend to be high in fat and have something which is tomato based. It can still have plenty of flavour, but reducing, the cream or cheese will help to keep the fat content down.

In the evening, you want to have something light which will keep you going through the night. Avoid cheese or nuts because they are hard to digest and can cause nightmares. A wholegrain cereal, wholemeal toast or wholegrain crackers could be a good choice. Some people prefer a milky drink.

What to Drink

It is important to drink regularly through the day as well. Try to avoid too much caffeine as this can make you feel stressed, although there has been research saying that it is healthy. |It may be something that you will need to judge yourself, depending on how you react to it.

Avoid high calorie drinks such as milk based drinks and sugary juices and fizzy drinks. It is better to drink water and tea with the occasional coffee. These days coffee and tea and mainly decaffeinated using the water method. This is a more natural process than the chemical processes that used to be used and so it is no longer an unhealthy choice. Try to only have one fruit juice a day as multiple juices do not count towards your five a day and they will add unnecessary calories. The acid in fruit juice and fizzy drinks can also damage your teeth.

Therefore aim to have a drink with every meal and some afterwards as well. Ideally a juice and coffee with breakfast, tea mid morning, water with lunch and tea afterwards, tea mid afternoon, water with the evening meal and coffee afterwards and then tea in the evening would be a typical pattern. Obviously you may prefer different types of drinks but this quantity would be ideal.

There used to be a lot of talk that the only think you needed was water and that other drinks didn't count towards your bodies need for liquid. However, there has been a new way of thinking that any fluids are good. This includes the fluid content of food as well as tea and coffee. However, caffeine can act as a diuretic and therefore make you need the loo more often. This means that if you have a lot of caffeinated drinks, then you may need to drink more.

Alcohol does not count towards your fluid intake. This really dehydrates the body and as it is very high in calories and is toxic too. It is a good idea to avoid it as much as you can or just stick to a small amount on the odd occasion. The worst thing you can do is to drink in large quantities, either all the time or on the odd occasion. It is very damaging for your body. There are recommendations that in order to give your liver time to recover form any sort of alcohol, you should have three days gap without drinking between every drinking session.

Listening to Your Body

One reason that certain diets do not work for us, could be because we are not listening to our body. If there was a diet that worked for everyone, then there would be no obesity, but this is not the case. However, some diets do seem to work for certain people. Why is that?

It could be that certain diets work for certain body types. We are all genetically different and the way that our bodies work are not all the same. You may think we are, but when you consider that some people are on medication because certain parts of their body are not working properly, then you can begin to understand that this could mean that we all have different needs.

For example, if we have diabetes, then we have to inject insulin and too much insulin can cause fat to form more easily in the body. If we are in pain, then we may find that we have no appetite. If we have just fought off some sort of infection, then we may need a boost in certain areas, to help the body to replenish itself.

Obviously, we do not all have a medical condition, but we do all differ in many ways and so even if we have excess adrenaline or hypoglycaemia, it may not have been diagnosed or even noticed, but it will have an effect on the body and its need for fuel.

This means that we may find that certain weight loss methods work better for us as individuals. For example, some people seem to lose weight, only if they are exercising and others find that exercise makes little difference but the food makes a big difference. It can be difficult to know whether this is really true, because not a lot of research has been done in this area. Also it is hard to control what people eat and how much exercise they do, without keeping them housed at a research laboratory for a significant period of time. Not only is that expensive, but it is also difficult to find anyone willing to take part. This is why experiments tend to be carried out on animals.

Although they can be controlled well and there have been great findings from them. They do not have the same sort of environment as us though. They do not have the stress of daily life, temptation with 'bad' foods, limited budget to spend on food, limited time for exercising etc. This means that it is not really possible to apply results of this sort of experiments to humans in a 'normal' situation.

There has been a very interesting experiment carried out by Christopher Gardner of Stamford University, where different diets were compared over an 18 month period. They didn't take participants in to a laboratory and feed them each day, they decided to teach them about a specific diet and ask them to stick to it as best they could. This was good, because it replicated the situation most people are in when on a diet. Not all of them stuck to the diet as would be expected in this sort of situation. They compared high carbohydrate, low carbohydrate and other diets to see which was most effective over the 18 months. They found that the low carbohydrate Atkins diet was best for losing weight. People lost more weight at the beginning more quickly and so on average there was more weight lost. However, just as many people had put on weight by the end of the study as with the other diets.

It was very interesting result and obviously gave no clues as to why this particular diet was better. The claims, by the author say that it fills you up more and that helps you stick to it. However, personally it might seem that because it includes a lot of foods that people really like, such as cream, fatty meats and butter plus not many foods they do not like, such as fruits and vegetables, it could be easier to stick to over a longer term. You do have to eliminate sugar and this could be difficult for some people. Of course it could be argued that it is more like our 'natural' diet which was meat and berries and things like that, but just because we used to eat that diet, it does not mean that it is a healthy diet for us today. What we do on a daily basis is very different, therefore our needs are different and we live a lot longer and have different diseases to fight.

There are also many people who have tried the Atkins diet and found that it has not worked for them. It is also something which is impossible for vegans and very difficult for vegetarians to stick to.

How To Move Forward

All this information could seem extremely confusing. No diet works in the long term, some work better than others in the short term and we need to have a healthy balanced diet with a good variety of food, but limiting out range of food stops us eating as much. It is all rather overwhelming!!

However, as mentioned earlier, it is a good idea to take small steps, making changes which you know you can keep up for life. You need to think about what you are eating and drinking and what exercise you are doing in order to find out where you need to make changes. It has been found that people always under report how much they eat. This is not always because they want to cheat, but very likely to be because they do not remember. However, try to be as honest as you can and then you have a better chance of being able to help yourself.

You need to think about exercise and food and how you are doing with each of them. If you do not exercise at all, then this could be the place to work on first. It can be difficult to find a way to fit exercising in to your daily routine and also to stick to it all of the time. Perhaps think about why you do not exercise and whether you can resolve that somehow. It might be because you do not have time or because you just do not like it. However, busy people who like exercise, find time for it and so it could be more to do with your dislike of it, when it comes down to it.

Eating can be much more complex. There are many people who are emotional eaters and either do not eat or eat a lot when they are stressed. Others eat very little and then binge because they are hungry or their blood sugar is low. Some just eat too much all the time. Others do not understand about calories and what is healthy and what is not.

This is why writing it down might help. You might be able to see patterns in your eating, perhaps a certain time of the day when you tend to be more unhealthy or a certain day of the week or even day in the month. You may even find when you visit certain places or are with certain people you tend to eat in a particular way.

Exercising

If you exercise regularly, then you may think that you do not need to do any more. If you do not exercise much, then you may not want to do any more. However, it is important to make sure that you do get enough exercise.

There has also been a research study where people who have lost a large amount of weight and kept it off for three years were asked what their diet secrets were. They all had different things that they did, but most of them exercised for at least an hour every day. This could indicate that exercise is something which can help with weight control. The study did not go in to detail as to what sort of exercise the people were doing.

Exercising can make you hungry, you burn off calories and perhaps fat and so your body will be asking you to replenish. Therefore it is not necessarily something that will help you lose weight, because you will want to eat more. However, it is essential to exercise, to stay healthy and so you should do it anyway.

Also if you time your exercise right, then you may not eat more. If you exercise before a meal, then just eat your normal amount, you should feel full up despite having exercised and will not end up eating more. You will also get used to it after a while.

It is good to try to focus on ways that you can do more exercise. Often we tend to find ways that we can avoid it, rather than do more. However, it can make a big difference and get you in to great new habits.

Some people do not like the thought of exercise but it does not have to mean sweating it out in the gym. You can do any sort of moving about at all. It can mean anything from walking to dancing. Even cleaning the house, washing the car and gardening burn off calories.

You will often find that people who are thin, tend to be constantly doing things, moving around the place and buzzing. People who are larger tend to do a desk job or sit in a car all day and they do not move unless they have to.

It is possible to change though. Once you start moving more, you will start to realise how good it can make you feel and you will want to do it more and more.

The great thing is that not only will you be burning calories and losing weight, you will be improving your muscle tone and the way your body looks. If you are getting out of breath, you will also be exercising your heart.

If there are particular parts of your body that you would like to shape up, you can do so by doing particular types of exercise that will work those muscles. It can be a great way to start feeling better about how you look and as you like how you look, you will feel more inspired to carry on with the exercise.

It is important to fit the exercise in to your daily routine. Make sure that you find a time that you can do it each day. You do not want any excuse to avoid doing it and so make sure that there is no way that this can happen.

You will need to be determined, but once you make it a habit, then it will be much easier to carry on with it.

Eating

It is a good idea to start to change your attitude towards food. Think about the purpose of eating and why your body needs you to do it. If you think of it more as a mechanical process, just something we do to survive, rather than a pleasurable experience, then this could help.

You need to stop treating yourself with food. If you have achieved something good then buy a magazines, book, item of clothing, jewellery or just give yourself a pat on the back. Food should never been seen as a reward, using it as such can cause all sorts of problems. It can be something that we have grown up with and we certainly don't want to pass the habit on to our own children.

Sometimes we get hormonal and feel the need to eat. Perhaps something sweet or salty or we just want to feel really full up. Some people feel that if we crave food in this way, then we should ignore the craving. Other people think that we should give in to it. It can be best to give in to it in moderation. That means have something sweet or salty but not too much of something or try to keep it as healthy as possible. If you try to resist temptation completely, you may find that you eventually end up eating much more than you were originally intending to anyway. You know your own body better than anyone else does. So think about your craving and whether it is better to ignore it or better to give in to it.

It is also worth thinking about whether the food is worth the calories. A healthy food item is always worth the calories but something unhealthy may not be. Think about the amount of pleasure you might get from the food and whether it is worth it in terms of how much weight you could put on and the damage that you might do to your body.

Stay Thin For Life by Rachel Henderson

It can be worth trying to think about something that could really inspire you to lose weight. Many people who lose lots of weight, find that something happens in their life which makes them want to lose weight. This could be a comment from someone, a health condition, the way they look or something else. You may have lost weight before and something like this could have been the reason, think back and see whether it can inspire you again. This time write it down and make sure that you continuously remind yourself of it.

If you have a family history of a certain disease, then it could be that the way you eat could effect your chances of getting it. This could certainly be something that could potentially inspire you to look after your body better. Imagine what it could be like if you have to manage when you are not healthy.

It could be a good idea to actually list down all the good reasons why you should change to a healthy diet and exercise more. Put the list somewhere visible so that you can use it to remind yourself of why you should not just be eating anything you like and you should be looking after yourself better.

Action Plan

It is important to therefore have an action plan. Start off by writing down lots of good reasons why you should lose weight. Then write down what you would like to achieve in terms of weight/size/clothes size and fitness levels. If you think it will help you, put a time scale down as well, perhaps in stages or just when you want to be at your target. Then write yourself a promise, that you will work as hard as you can to achieve that target.

Now you have to start working on it. Hopefully you have already started thinking about what form of exercise you want to do. Think at what time of day you feel that you could fit it in as well. Then think about what type of exercise you want to do. It can be a good idea to build up slowly and do not commit to doing too much. If you overdo things, you will get exhausted and not be able to sustain it. You could write yourself out a plan where you work out how long it will take to build up the exercise you are doing to a level that you will be happy with. This could be over a very long time period or a relatively short one. It all depends on your current fitness levels and how much exercise you want to do.

The eating needs a similar approach. Work out how much you want to reduce your eating by, perhaps by quantity or calories or perhaps by cutting out particular foods. Work out how you can reduce it all slowly so that you will be able to sustain the changes. There are lots of small changes that you can make which could add up to a big difference. Here is a list to start you off:

Take stairs instead of lifts or escalators

Get off the bus a stop early or park the furthest you can from the door

Start taking regular walks

Stay Thin For Life by Rachel Henderson

Join up to an exercise class

Get an exercise machine to use at home

Look at exercise DVD's and see if there are any you like

Do more exercise based console games

Start walking a little bit faster

Get a pet dog so you have to walk twice a day

Change from buying whole milk, to semi-skimmed milk

Have skinny lattes and cappuccinos rather than normal ones

Choose lower calorie chocolate bars and eat them less often

Limit how many cakes/biscuits you have each week

Put less food on your plate or use a smaller plate

Replace some of your unhealthy foods with fruit and vegetables

Try out some new, lower fat recipes

Investigate healthier options when you eat out

Cook more at home, rather than eating out or buying ready meals

Limit how many take aways you have

Swap high fat cheese to a lower fat sort

Replace cream with yoghurt

Stay Thin For Life by Rachel Henderson

Use less butter

Bake less often

Replace puddings with fruit or yoghurt or cut them out

Eat until you are not hungry, rather than until you are full

Remember that you can always go back for more, there is no need to overfill your plate

Limit unhealthy choices to once a day and maybe once a week eventually

Avoid walking past shops where you buy unhealthy things

Never go out shopping hungry or else you will buy more unhealthy things

Avoid buying food that tempt you to overeat

Slowly build up the changes that you are making so that you do not get completely overwhelmed by everything. Even if you are only making one change a month, it is better than making no changes at all. Just make sure that you are fully committed to those changes and that you know that you will stick with them.

If you do find that you do not stick with what you have resolved to do, then do not give up completely. Just move on from it and go back to eating more healthily again. It can be tricky, there are temptations all around us and so it can be difficult to resist things all of the time.

Do not lose hope, just understand that we all make mistakes and that we should not see a set back as a big failure. Just realise that it happened, but it will not continue to happen, day after day.

Stay Thin For Life by Rachel Henderson

Sometimes we cannot help being unhealthy. If we are at someone else's house and served food, we have to eat what we are given and so this could mean that we have a set back without it being our fault. Just be polite and eat what you are given, enjoy the food but know that you will go back to your healthy ways, as soon as you can.

Eating and Stress

When we are stressed some people eat more and some people eat less. We all deal with it in different ways. Some of us will also tend to gain weight and others lose it. This is not always linked with what we eat, it does seem that the body can be prone to holding on to fat reserves when we are stressed and so even if we do not eat much, we do not lose weight and it can be easy to put it on.

Stress is a reaction to a situation that we cannot cope well with. It can be anything and it varies form person to person. Some people enjoy an adrenalin buzz and something which might be perceived as stressful to some people is not to others. So don't label certain situations as stressful, it is actually anything that you personally find that you cannot cope with, that would be considered to be stressful to you.

It is a good idea to work hard to manage stress. A healthy balanced diet can help with this, especially if your stress is related to your blood sugar levels as cutting out pure forms of sugar will help to balance blood sugar. Relaxation exercises can also be good as can meditation. Even taking a bath or doing something distracting like watching your favourite television program can help to reduce stress levels. It is good to try to find something that you find works for you.If you eat as a reaction to stress, then try to be aware of it. See whether you can reduce your stress in a different way, rather than eating. If you stop eating because of stress, then it is a good idea to try to have something. You will be deprived of nutrients otherwise and this will not be good for you. It may also mean that you will be more likely to binge, when you do decide to start eating again. Also, your body will hold on to all the fat that it can, because it will panic that you will be starving it. So when you start eating again, you will find that it is all stored as energy.

Weight and sleep

Getting a good nights sleep is important to the body. There are many health benefits as it is the time when the body repairs itself. Although not everyone seems to need the same amount of sleep, it is recommended that most people should have 8 hours a night. If you do not normally sleep this amount, then it could be worth trying for a week and seeing if it makes a difference.

A lack of sleep can obviously make us feel tired. When we are tired we tend to want to eat food, to give us an energy boost. This does not work, because it is sleep that we need. Therefore it can be tempting to keep eating and eating and this can cause weight gain. With severe tiredness, you may not even notice how much you are eating, until it is too late.

Going to bed early can even be a way of eating less. If you are hungry in the evening, then going to bed may stop you from eating extra.

Some people find that they do not sleep well and they wake up in the middle of the night and get food. It is often said that eating at night is the worst thing to do because you do not use up any of the energy. However, if you are exercising, then you will be burning off fat, as a result of that exercise for up to 12 hours afterwards and so this may not necessarily be true. However, if you are eating in the night it could be meaning you are taking in too many calories. It is a good idea to try to find out why you eat in the night and whether you can do something else instead. It could be due to sleeping problems, which might need to be addressed by your doctor. It could be because it is a habit which you need to break.

If your blood sugar crashes in the night, it can mean that you have difficulty sleeping and you could have nightmares and then wake up unable to get back to sleep. However, if you eat a good diet, then your blood sugar should be more balanced and hopefully your sleep will be improved as a result.

Weight and the Weather

When the weather gets cold we often start to feel like having lots of stodgy carbohydrates like pastries and pies and mashed potato. These can be high in calories. However, it does use extra energy to keep us warm and so we may be burning off calories this way. It is worth listening to your body, but not overeating too much so that you put on weight. Use a sensible approach.

In the summer you may not feel like eating so much, especially if it is very warm. However, do not fill up on high calorie drinks. It is sensible to drink more, but try to go for lower calorie option such as water. Fizzy drinks with lots of sugar or sweetener are not such a healthy option. Fruit juice may seem better but the high acidity can be bad for the teeth.

As the winter starts we get tempted to think about weight loss because of looking good at Christmas. In the summer, there is the worry of wearing a bikini on holiday. However, associating these times of year with a diet could be a big problem. Our body may start to worry that it will be starved of food or nutrients and may start to hold on to fat because of it. It is better to just approach each time of the year with the same attitude really. Perhaps having more hot meals in the winter, soups instead of salads and hot drinks instead of cold ones and then cooling down in the winter with iced drinks and refrigerated foods.

Trying to hep your body with cooling or heating can help to balance the energy levels. If your body is working hard to keep warm or cool, then you may feel hungry because you need the energy and so by being in tune with your body and eating what it needs, you can do better.

Getting Support

When we are making big life changes, it can be very important to make sure that we get the support that we need from those around us. If you normally have someone cook your meals for you, then it might be difficult to convince them to change what you are eating, especially if it makes things difficult for them. You may also find that you need their help, to keep you sticking at things.

Do not be afraid to ask for help. It can be difficult, when you are in a close relationship, if you ask someone to help you lose weight though. At times of weakness, they may try to encourage you to take the healthy option and it is possible for you to see it as a criticism of your behaviour or even of how you look. Therefore think hard about the consequences of asking for help and whether it might be best not to. It could just be a case of making sure that you discuss things through thoroughly with the people you do ask to help you and make sure that you all understand how tough things might be and how it might be possible that you could react badly to one another at times.

It can be easier to make changes with someone else though. It can be worth considering working together with someone. If they are doing well with things, then it can encourage you and vice versa. As long as you do not encourage each other to not stick to things, then it can really help. Many people find a lot of benefit from being with others who have similar goals to them and that is why slimming clubs are so popular. You could consider joining one or you could just work on a personal basis with someone that you know.

Your Family

Most people live with their family. Dieting can be a very difficult thing to do with family around. But making healthy food choices is much easier. This is because the food is healthy and good for everyone, which means that you can feed them the same food as you.

It is good to be able to do this because not only does it make things easier for you and make it a lot easier for you to stick to eating a healthy diet, it also means that you will be making them healthier as well.

It is so important to make sure that you give children all the right food messages when you are bringing them up. This means that you feed them healthily and help them to understand why eating healthily is so important. They will also grow up being more healthy and less likely to pick up any nasty illnesses. Hopefully the eating habits you form with them as children will continue as they get older.

Temptation

There is temptation all around us, all of the time. Even if we only keep healthy foods in the house, there are always things to tempt us when we are shopping, having a drink out or when we visit others. Sometimes it can be very difficult to resist temptation.

We cannot avoid temptation because it will always be there somewhere. We can do things to keep it out of our sight at home perhaps, but when we visit friends and family or go out and about, you will always see tempting things around. It is therefore important to find a way of coping with this.

The thing is that if we continuously deprive ourselves of the things that we really like, then we will not feel good. This can be one reason that people move away from healthy eating. They decide that they deserve to have the tasty alternatives, that they have so many happy memories associated with. However, it is important to keep thinking to yourself that you are deserving.

You deserve to be healthy and feel good and you will only achieve that by eating well. You do not 'deserve' those unhealthy foods. They will only make you feel guilty and not like the way that you look. They will also cause you get unwell and have a poor quality of life. So decide that you deserve to be healthy, you deserve to have a good quality of life. You want to live a long and happy life, watch your grandchildren grow up and you deserve to be fit and healthy and to look good. You want to feel good about every aspect of yourself and how you look can be a big part in this.

So when you are tempted to eat something that is not healthy, think about what you deserve. How hard you have worked and how much better you will be, both in how you look and feel and your health, if you take the healthy rather than unhealthy option.

Positive Thinking

It is really important to have the right attitude towards your healthier lifestyle. You need to understand that unless you know that you can be strong and fully committed then things may not be successful for you. It is important to be positive that things will work for you.

It is a good idea to write down the advantages of you being healthier and look at this every day. This will help to motivate you to succeed. If you keep thinking about the future and how things will be then, how much healthier and fitter you will be, how different you will look and how this will effect your life overall.

It is good to focus on this every day, not just on the days when things have not gone as well as you had hoped. This should help you to focus, when you are tempted to not be healthy. When you want to overeat or eat unhealthy foods or when you want to skip your exercise session for that day. Focus on why you are working hard and what the rewards will be for you.

It can also be good to reward yourself at certain milestones. Buy yourself a book or magazine or a new outfit. Something that is not food related but will make you feel happy. Se it to reward yourself in a way that is meaningful to you. This could be for a certain amount of weight loss or it could be for inches lost. It might be for reaching an exercise target, perhaps running a race or doing a certain amount of gym sessions. Think of something that will mean something to you and a reward which will also be good for you.

Feeling happy is important to all of us. If you have previously found pleasure form food, then you need to find it elsewhere. Hopefully you will find it in exercising, but it may not be this.

Find something to do that you enjoy, that you can do instead of eating, even do it when you are tempted to eat. Only you know what you enjoy and so it will be up to you to find that thing which suits you the best.

Conclusion

Getting healthy is not always easy. However, you need to get yourself in to the right mind set. Be determined to succeed, understand the benefits and the rewards for doing so and this will help you be able to get yourself prepared for some life changing decisions. Think about your way of life, how much your exercise and how you eat and how you can change those so you are a healthier person. Good health has great results and you will also feel better about how you look, have more energy and generally a better all round approach to life. It can only do you good, so why not give it a try. Step by step, you will be able to change your bad habits in to good ones and lose that excess fat and become a healthier person as a result.

Good luck.

Printed in Great Britain
by Amazon

36081522R00030